AGELESS IN THE 50s:

The Ultimate Guide For Women Over 50 to Look and Feel Their Best

By

Jane Gain

Introduction

Chapter 1: Understanding Women Over 50
and Their Nutritional Needs

- Metabolic changes that occur with
  age
- Hormonal changes and how they
  affect weight loss
- Nutritional requirements for women
  over 50

Chapter 2: The Science Behind Intermittent
Fasting

- Different types of intermittent fasting
- The benefits of intermittent fasting
  for women over 50
- The risks and precautions to consider

Chapter 3: Getting Started with Intermittent
Fasting

- How to prepare for intermittent fasting
- Tips for making the transition easier
- Common mistakes to avoid

Chapter 4: Intermittent Fasting Strategies for Women Over 50

Chapter 5: Maximizing the Benefits of Intermittent Fasting
- Exercise and intermittent fasting
- Meal planning and nutrient-dense foods
- Stress management and intermittent fasting

Chapter 6: A 28 days meal Plan

Chapter 7: Frequently Asked Questions About Intermittent Fasting for Women Over 50

Chapter 8: Conclusion

Introduction

Intermittent fasting has become increasingly popular in recent years as a way to improve overall health and promote weight loss. But what exactly is intermittent fasting, and how does it work?

Intermittent fasting is an eating pattern that involves alternating periods of fasting and eating. Unlike traditional diets that restrict calories every day, intermittent fasting allows individuals to consume their usual calorie intake within a certain window of time, typically ranging from a few hours to several days.

The benefits of intermittent fasting extend beyond weight loss. Studies have shown that it can improve insulin sensitivity, reduce inflammation, promote cellular repair, and even increase lifespan. It has also been linked to a lower risk of chronic diseases such as heart disease, diabetes, and certain types of cancer.

In this book, we will explore the science behind intermittent fasting and how it can be used to promote overall health and well-being. We will also provide practical tips and strategies for getting started with intermittent fasting, maximizing its benefits, and addressing common concerns and questions. Whether you're looking to lose weight, improve your health, or simply want to try a new approach to eating, this book will serve as your comprehensive guide to intermittent fasting.

Chapter 1

Understanding Women Over 50 and Their Nutritional Needs

Intermittent fasting is an eating pattern that involves alternating periods of eating and fasting. It does not necessarily restrict the types or amounts of foods consumed, but rather the timing of meals.

There are different approaches to intermittent fasting, but the most common ones include time-restricted feeding, where individuals eat within a specific window of time each day (such as an 8-hour eating window), and alternate-day fasting, where individuals alternate between days of eating normally and days of consuming very few calories.

Intermittent fasting has gained popularity as a potential way to promote weight loss and improve overall health. It has been linked to benefits such as improved insulin sensitivity, reduced inflammation, and a lower risk of chronic diseases like heart disease, diabetes, and certain types of cancer.

While intermittent fasting may not be suitable for everyone, it can be a flexible and sustainable approach to healthy eating for many individuals.

☐ How Hormonal and Metabolic Changes Affect Weight Loss

- **Slower Metabolism**

As women age, their metabolism may slow down, resulting in fewer calories burned at rest. This can make it more difficult to lose weight and easier to gain weight.

- **Insulin resistance**

Age-related insulin resistance can lead to weight gain and difficulty losing weight. This is because insulin is responsible for regulating blood sugar levels, and when the body becomes resistant to insulin, it can lead to an increased appetite and weight gain.

- **Leptin resistance**

Age-related leptin resistance can lead to overeating and weight gain. This is because leptin is responsible for regulating hunger and metabolism, and when the body becomes resistant to leptin, it can lead to an increased appetite and weight gain.

- **Estrogen levels**

During menopause, changes in estrogen levels can lead to weight gain and difficulty losing weight in women. This is because estrogen plays a role in regulating metabolism and body fat distribution.

- **Thyroid hormones**

Changes in thyroid hormone levels can also affect weight loss in women over 50. An underactive thyroid can lead to a slower metabolism and weight gain, while an overactive thyroid can lead to a faster metabolism and weight loss.

- **Cortisol**

Age-related changes in cortisol levels can lead to weight gain, particularly in the abdominal area. This is because cortisol is responsible for regulating stress and can lead to increased weight gain when levels are high.

☐ Nutritional Requirements For Women Over 50

Nutritional requirements for women over 50 can differ from those of younger women due to changes in metabolism and hormonal levels. Here are some important nutritional requirements for women over 50:

- **Protein**

Protein is important for maintaining muscle mass and bone health, which can decline with age. Women over 50 should aim for at least 1 gram of protein per kilogram of body weight per day.

- **Calcium and Vitamin D**

These nutrients are important for maintaining bone health and preventing osteoporosis. Women over 50 should aim for 1200 milligrams of calcium per day and 600-800 international units (IU) of vitamin D per day.

- **Fiber**

Adequate fiber intake can help with digestion and reduce the risk of chronic diseases. Women over 50 should aim for at least 21 grams of fiber per day.

- **Omega-3 Fatty Acids**

These healthy fats can help with brain function, heart health, and inflammation. Women over 50 should aim for at least 1-2 servings of fatty fish per week or consider taking a fish oil supplement.

- **Vitamin B12**

As we age, our bodies may have more difficulty absorbing vitamin B12 from food. Women over 50 should aim for at least 2.4 micrograms of vitamin B12 per day.

Water

Staying hydrated is important for overall health, especially as we age. Women over 50 should aim for at least 8-10 cups of water per day.

Chapter 2

The Science Behind Intermittent Fasting

☐ Types Of Intermittent Fasting

There are several different types of intermittent fasting, including:

- **Time-Restricted Feeding**

This involves eating during a specific time window each day and fasting for the remaining hours. For example, a common time-restricted feeding schedule is 16:8, where one fast for 16 hours and eats during an 8-hour window.

- **Alternate-Day Fasting**

This involves fasting every other day, where one eats normally on non-fasting days and consumes only a small amount of food or fasts completely on fasting days.

- **5:2 Diet**

This involves consuming a regular diet for five days per week and consuming only 500-600 calories on two non-consecutive days of the week.

- **Eat-Stop-Eat**

This involves fasting for 24 hours once or twice per week and eating normally on non-fasting days.

- **The Warrior Diet**

This involves consuming one large meal at night and fasting during the day.

- **Spontaneous Meal Skipping**

This involves skipping meals when not hungry or when it is not convenient to eat, and listening to one's body's hunger signals.

☐ Benefits Of Intermittent Fasting For Women Over 50

Intermittent fasting can offer several benefits for women over 50, including:

- **Weight Loss**

Intermittent fasting can help women over 50 loose weight by reducing calorie intake and increasing fat burning.

- **Improved Metabolism**

Intermittent fasting can help improve metabolic function by reducing insulin resistance and increasing growth hormone levels.

- **Reduced Inflammation**

Intermittent fasting can help reduce inflammation in the body, which is a risk factor for many chronic diseases.

- **Improved Brain Function**

Intermittent fasting may help improve cognitive function and reduce the risk of neurodegenerative diseases.

- **Lowered Risk of Chronic Diseases**

Intermittent fasting can help reduce the risk of chronic diseases such as heart disease, diabetes, and cancer.

Improved Sleep: Intermittent fasting can improve sleep quality by regulating circadian rhythms and increasing melatonin production.

Increased Longevity: Intermittent fasting has been shown to increase lifespan and improve overall healthspan in animal studies, although more research is needed to confirm these findings in humans.

☐ The Risks And Precautions To Consider

While intermittent fasting can offer several potential health benefits, it may not be suitable for everyone. Here are some risks and precautions to consider:

- **Nutrient deficiencies**

Depending on the type of intermittent fasting, it may be difficult to consume all necessary nutrients within the limited eating window. It is important to ensure that meals are nutrient-dense and balanced to avoid nutrient deficiencies.

- **Dehydration**

Prolonged fasting periods can lead to dehydration. It is important to stay hydrated during fasting periods by drinking plenty of water and other fluids.

- **Blood sugar fluctuations**

Intermittent fasting can lead to blood sugar fluctuations, which can be problematic for individuals with diabetes or other blood sugar issues. It is important to monitor blood sugar levels closely and consult with a healthcare provider before starting an intermittent fasting program.

- **Increased hunger and cravings**

Some individuals may experience increased hunger and cravings during fasting periods, which can make it difficult to stick to the program. It is important to listen to the body's hunger signals and consume enough calories and nutrients during the eating window.

- **Medication interactions**

Intermittent fasting can interact with certain medications, such as blood pressure medications or medications that require food intake. It is important to consult with a healthcare provider before starting an intermittent fasting program if taking any medications.

- **Eating disorders**

Individuals with a history of eating disorders may be more susceptible to developing disordered eating patterns with intermittent fasting. It is important to consult with a healthcare provider or therapist before starting an intermittent fasting program if having a history of disordered eating.

Pregnancy or breastfeeding: Intermittent fasting is not recommended for pregnant or breastfeeding women as it can affect nutrient intake and potentially harm the developing baby.

Chapter 3

Getting Started with Intermittent Fasting

☐ How To Prepare For Intermittent Fasting

Preparing for intermittent fasting can help you have a successful experience. Here are some tips to prepare for intermittent fasting:

Consult with your healthcare provider: Before starting any new dietary pattern, it is important to consult with your healthcare provider to make sure it is safe for you.

- **Choose a fasting method**

There are many different methods of intermittent fasting, so choose one that fits your lifestyle and preferences.

- **Gradually adjust your eating pattern**

If you are used to eating three meals a day, try gradually reducing it to two meals a day before starting intermittent fasting. This can help your body adjust to the new eating pattern.

- **Plan your meals**

When you are not fasting, plan your meals to make sure you are getting enough nutrients and calories to sustain your body.

- **Stay hydrated**

During fasting periods, make sure you drink enough water to stay hydrated. This can help reduce hunger and keep your body functioning properly.

Stock up on healthy snacks

When you are not fasting, stock up on healthy snacks such as fruits, vegetables, and nuts to help you get through fasting periods.

Manage stress

Stress can lead to overeating, so it is important to find ways to manage stress during both eating and fasting periods.

By following these tips, you can prepare yourself for a successful experience with intermittent fasting.

☐ Tips For Making The Transition Easier

Transitioning to intermittent fasting can be challenging, but some tips can help make the process easier:

- **Start gradually**

If you are new to fasting, start with a shorter fasting period and gradually increase the duration over time. This can help your body adjust to the new eating pattern.

- **Keep busy**

During fasting periods, keep yourself busy with activities such as reading, exercising, or spending time with friends to help take your mind off of food.

- **Stay hydrated**

Drinking plenty of water during fasting periods can help reduce hunger and keep your body functioning properly.

- **Eat high-fiber foods**

High-fiber foods such as fruits, vegetables, and whole grains can help you feel fuller for longer and reduce cravings during fasting periods.

- **Get enough sleep**

Getting enough sleep can help regulate hormones that control hunger and appetite, making it easier to stick to the fasting schedule.

- **Be mindful of what you eat**

During eating periods, choose nutrient-dense foods that will provide your body with the energy it needs to function properly.

- **Be patient**

It may take some time for your body to adjust to the new eating pattern, so be patient and stick with it.

By following these tips, you can make the transition to intermittent fasting easier and more successful.

☐ Common Mistakes To Avoid

Here are some common mistakes to avoid when practicing intermittent fasting:

- **Eating too much during eating periods**

It can be tempting to overeat during eating periods, but this can negate the benefits of fasting. Stick to a healthy, balanced diet during eating periods.

- **Not drinking enough water**

Staying hydrated is important during fasting periods. Make sure to drink plenty of water throughout the day.

- **Not getting enough sleep**

Lack of sleep can increase hunger and affect hormone levels, making it more difficult to stick to the fasting schedule.

- **Fasting for too long**

It is important to choose a fasting method that is safe and sustainable for you. Fasting for too long can be harmful to your health.

- **Not seeking medical advice**

It is important to consult with your healthcare provider before starting intermittent fasting, especially if you have any underlying health conditions or are taking medications.

- **Not listening to your body**

Pay attention to how your body feels during fasting periods. If you feel lightheaded or dizzy, it may be time to break your fast.

- **Giving up too quickly**

It can take some time for your body to adjust to intermittent fasting. Stick with it and be patient.

By avoiding these common mistakes, you can have a successful experience with intermittent fasting.

Chapter 4

Intermittent Fasting Strategies For Women Over 50

- **Plan your workouts**

Plan your workouts during eating periods when you have more energy and can properly fuel your body. Avoid intense workouts during fasting periods as they may lead to fatigue and decrease performance.

- **Listen to your body**

If you feel tired or lightheaded during exercise while fasting, stop and break your fast to properly fuel your body. Overexerting yourself during a fast can be dangerous and counterproductive.

- **Consider low-intensity exercises**

Low-intensity exercises such as walking, yoga, or stretching can be beneficial during fasting periods and can help reduce stress.

- **Avoid overeating after exercise**

It can be tempting to overeat after a workout, especially during eating periods. However, it's important to stick to a balanced diet and avoid overeating to avoid negating the benefits of intermittent fasting.

Chapter 5

Maximizing The Benefits Of Intermittent Fasting

☐ Meal Planning And Nutrient-dense Foods

Meal planning is an important aspect of intermittent fasting, and it's important to focus on nutrient-dense foods that provide your body with the nutrients it needs to function properly. Here are some tips for meal planning and choosing nutrient-dense foods:

- **Plan ahead**

Plan your meals and snacks to make sure you have healthy options on hand during eating periods.

- **Choose nutrient-dense foods**

Focus on foods that are high in nutrients such as fruits, vegetables, lean proteins, and whole grains. These foods will provide your body with the energy it needs and help you feel fuller for longer.

- **Include healthy fats**

Healthy fats such as avocado, nuts, and olive oil can help keep you feeling full and provide your body with essential nutrients.

- **Avoid processed foods**

Processed foods are often high in calories, sugar, and unhealthy fats, and can sabotage your weight loss goals. Choose whole foods whenever possible.

- **Be mindful of portion sizes**

Even healthy foods can lead to weight gain if you eat too much. Be mindful of portion sizes and pay attention to your body's hunger and fullness cues.

By focusing on nutrient-dense foods and planning your meals, you can make the most of your eating periods during intermittent fasting and support your overall health and weight loss goals.

☐ Exercise And Intermittent Fasting

Exercise can be a great addition to intermittent fasting and can help you achieve your health and fitness goals. Here are some things to consider when combining exercise with intermittent fasting:

- **Stay hydrated**

Make sure to drink plenty of water before, during, and after your workouts, especially if you are fasting. Dehydration can lead to fatigue, cramps, and other negative side effects.

- **Plan your workouts**

Plan your workouts during eating periods when you have more energy and can properly fuel your body. Avoid intense workouts during fasting periods as they may lead to fatigue and decrease performance.

- **Listen to your body**

If you feel tired or lightheaded during exercise while fasting, stop and break your fast to properly fuel your body. Overexerting yourself during a fast can be dangerous and counterproductive.

- **Consider low-intensity exercises**

Low-intensity exercises such as walking, yoga, or stretching can be beneficial during fasting periods and can help reduce stress.

- **Avoid overeating after exercise**

It can be tempting to overeat after a workout, especially during eating periods. However, it's important to stick to a balanced diet and avoid overeating to avoid negating the benefits of intermittent fasting.

Chapter 6

A 28 days meal plan

Sure, there's a 28-day meal plan for intermittent fasting for women over 50:

First, let's go over thc basics of intermittent fasting. There are several different approaches to intermittent fasting, but one popular method is the 16:8 method, which involves fasting for 16 hours and eating during an 8-hour window each day. For example, you might eat all of your meals between 12 pm and 8 pm and fast for the remaining 16 hours.

It's important to note that you should consult with your doctor before starting any new diet or exercise program, especially if you have any medical conditions or take any medications.

Here's a sample 28-day meal plan for intermittent fasting:

Day 1:

Lunch: Grilled chicken breast with roasted vegetables (zucchini, peppers, onions) and quinoa.

Dinner: Baked salmon with steamed broccoli and sweet potato.

Day 2:

Lunch: Greek salad with chicken (romaine lettuce, cucumber, tomato, olives, feta cheese, red onion, chicken) with olive oil and vinegar dressing.

Dinner: Stir-fried beef and vegetables (broccoli, mushrooms, peppers, onions) with brown rice.

Day 3:

Lunch: Tuna salad (tuna, mixed greens, cherry tomatoes, cucumber, red onion, avocado) with lemon vinaigrette.

Dinner: Baked chicken thighs with roasted Brussels sprouts and brown rice.

Day 4:

Lunch: Vegetable omelet (spinach, mushrooms, onions, bell peppers) with whole-grain toast.

Dinner: Grilled shrimp skewers with grilled asparagus and wild rice.

Day 5:

Lunch: Chickpea and vegetable curry (chickpeas, cauliflower, carrots, onions, garlic, ginger, tomato sauce, coconut milk) with brown rice.

Dinner: Grilled pork tenderloin with roasted sweet potatoes and green beans.

Day 6:

Lunch: Grilled chicken salad (mixed greens, tomatoes, cucumbers, shredded carrots, grilled chicken) with balsamic vinaigrette.

Dinner: Baked salmon with roasted Brussels sprouts and quinoa.

Day 7:

Lunch: Lentil soup with a side of mixed greens salad (mixed greens, cherry tomatoes, cucumber, red onion) with lemon vinaigrette.

Dinner: Grilled steak with roasted vegetables (broccoli, mushrooms, onions) and mashed sweet potatoes.

For the remaining 21 days, you can mix and match these meal ideas or come up with your own. Remember to stick to your 8-hour eating window and stay hydrated throughout the day. You may also want to consider incorporating low-intensity exercises, such as walking or yoga, into your daily routine.

Chapter 7

Frequently Asked Questions About Intermittent Fasting for Women Over 50

Here are some frequently asked questions about intermittent fasting for women over 50:

- **Is intermittent fasting safe for women over 50?**

Yes, intermittent fasting can be safe for women over 50 as long as it is done properly and with consideration of any underlying health conditions.

- **Can intermittent fasting help with weight loss for women over 50?**

Yes, intermittent fasting can be an effective weight loss tool for women over 50 as it helps to create a calorie deficit and can improve metabolic function.

- **What are some common types of intermittent fasting?**

Some common types of intermittent fasting include the 16/8 method, where you fast for 16 hours and eat during an 8-hour window, the 5:2 diet, where you eat normally for 5 days and restrict calories for 2 days, and alternate-day fasting, where you alternate between days of normal eating and restricted calorie intake.

- **Can I still exercise while intermittent fasting?**

Yes, it is possible to exercise while intermittent fasting, but it's important to schedule your workouts during eating periods when you have more energy and fuel for your body.

- **What are some nutrient-dense foods that can be eaten during eating periods?**

Nutrient-dense foods that can be eaten during eating periods include fruits, vegetables, lean proteins, whole grains, and healthy fats such as avocado, nuts, and olive oil.

- **Is it normal to feel hungry during fasting periods?**

Yes, it's normal to feel hungry during fasting periods, especially at the beginning. However, hunger pangs usually subside after the body adjusts to the new eating schedule.

- **Are there any risks associated with intermittent fasting?**

Intermittent fasting can pose risks for certain individuals with underlying health conditions, such as diabetes or eating disorders. It's important to consult with a healthcare provider before starting any new diet or exercise program.

Chapter 8

Conclusion

One of the benefits of intermittent fasting is that it is a flexible approach that can be customized to meet individual needs and preferences. There are several different types of intermittent fastings, such as the 16/8 method or alternate-day fasting, which can be adjusted based on personal goals and lifestyle.

However, it is important to note that intermittent fasting is not a magic solution or a one-size-fits-all approach. It requires patience, persistence, and a commitment to making lifestyle changes. It is also important to avoid common mistakes and take precautions to prevent potential risks.

Overall, with the right approach, intermittent fasting can be a powerful tool for women over

50 to improve their health and well-being. By listening to their bodies, making adjustments as needed, and seeking guidance from a healthcare professional, women can successfully incorporate intermittent fasting into their lifestyle and reap the benefits for years to come.